CONTENTS

IIFYM SNACKS

THE MACRO BLUEPRINT: NOURISHING YOUR WAY TO HEALTH WITH IIFYM AND RECIPES FOR SUCCESS

Welcome to "The Macro Blueprint: Nourishing Your Way to Health with IIFYM and Recipes for Success." In this comprehensive guide, you will learn about the revolutionary approach to dieting known as IIFYM, which stands for "If It Fits Your Macros." Here, we debunk the myth that eating healthily requires extreme sacrifices and instead introduce a novel way of achieving your fitness goals while still enjoying eating what you love. With this book, you will embark on a journey that forever changes your perception of dieting and health.

The IIFYM approach is as liberating as it is empowering. Rather than focusing solely on calorie counts, IIFYM promotes a balance of macronutrients - proteins, carbohydrates, and fats - tailored to your unique needs and objectives. Instead of shunning entire food groups or succumbing to a cycle of restriction and bingeing, IIFYM teaches you to use food as fuel, providing the nourishment your body requires to perform at its best.

The first part of this book will familiarize you with the principles of IIFYM. It demystifies macronutrients, discusses how to calculate your daily needs, and explains how to use these calculations to achieve your goals, whether they involve losing weight, building muscle, or maintaining a healthy lifestyle. From understanding your body's metabolic rate to fine-tuning the perfect macro balance, you'll become your own best nutritionist.

But this book is more than a guide to understanding IIFYM; it is also a cookbook filled with delicious, macro-friendly recipes that cater to a myriad of dietary preferences and needs. Each recipe includes a full macronutrient breakdown, making it easy for you to incorporate them into your daily plan. They are proof that healthy eating doesn't have to be bland or boring. From breakfast to dinner, vegetarian options to seafood delights, you'll discover a world of flavors while adhering to your macro goals.

The key to this approach is flexibility, meaning no food is off-limits as long as it fits within your macro allowances. This freedom can make dieting feel less like a chore and more like an exploration of personal nutrition, breaking the notion that you must deprive yourself to maintain a healthy lifestyle.

"The Macro Blueprint" is more than just a book; it's a pathway to sustainable health and fitness. By the end, you'll have the knowledge and tools you need to not only understand the IIFYM approach but also apply it to your everyday life.

Eating healthily should not be a struggle, but a joyful journey of self-discovery. So, let's leave the era of restrictive diets behind and step into a new age of balanced, macro-based nutrition. Welcome to IIFYM, your route to a healthier, happier you.

CHAPTER 1: UNDERSTANDING IIFYM – YOUR ROUTE TO BALANCED NUTRITION

Welcome to your first step in understanding "If It Fits Your Macros" (IIFYM) or the "flexible dieting" approach. This revolutionary concept eschews traditional restrictive diets in favor of a more balanced, flexible outlook on nutrition.

What Is IIFYM?

At its core, IIFYM is about balance. Rather than viewing food as "good" or "bad", it looks at the macronutrients—proteins, carbohydrates, and fats—that food contains. These macronutrients, often referred to as 'macros,' are the basic building blocks your body needs to function effectively.

Here's a brief overview of each macro's role:

- **Proteins** are essential for repairing and building body tissues, including muscles. They are also necessary for the production of enzymes and hormones.

- **Carbohydrates** are your body's primary energy source, fueling everything from your brain to your muscles during a workout.

- **Fats** are essential for many body functions, including nutrient absorption, hormone production, and maintaining body temperature. Despite the bad reputation, fats are crucial for overall health.

Calculating Your Macros

The heart of IIFYM is calculating the optimal balance of these macronutrients for your unique needs. This balance depends on several factors, including your age, gender, weight, activity level, and personal goals (e.g., weight loss, muscle gain, or maintenance).

There are many online calculators and mobile apps to help you determine your macros, but here's a basic overview of how it works:

1. Calculate your Basal Metabolic Rate (BMR) – This

is the amount of energy your body needs to perform basic functions like breathing and circulation at rest.

2. Determine your Total Daily Energy Expenditure (TDEE) – Multiply your BMR by an activity factor (which ranges from 1.2 for sedentary individuals to 2.5 for extremely active individuals) to account for the calories you burn through daily activities and exercise.

3. Set your macro ratios according to your goals – Once you know your TDEE, you can divide it into macronutrients. A common macro ratio is 40% carbohydrates, 30% proteins, and 30% fats, but this can be adjusted based on your individual needs and goals.

Applying IIFYM to Your Diet

Once you know your macro targets, the next step is to begin tracking your daily food intake to ensure you're meeting these goals. There are many food tracking apps available to help you log what you eat and see how it fits into your macro allowance.

One key principle of IIFYM is that no food is off-limits as long as it fits within your macro goals. This flexibility can make dieting more sustainable and enjoyable. However, it's still essential to prioritize nutrient-dense foods to meet your micronutrient needs and maintain overall health.

IIFYM is about giving you the tools to understand

how different foods impact your body and achieve your health goals in a flexible, sustainable way. You can still enjoy your favorite foods, but you'll learn how to balance them with other nutrients to fuel your body effectively.

As you progress through this book, you'll learn more about how to fine-tune your macro ratios, adjust your diet based on your progress, and incorporate a wide variety of foods to meet your macro goals. Together, we'll make your journey to health enjoyable and sustainable.

Remember, IIFYM is not just a diet—it's a lifestyle. It's about empowering you to understand your body's nutritional needs, taking control of your health, and enjoying the foods you love along the way. Let's take the next step in this exciting journey.

CHAPTER 2: MASTERING YOUR METABOLISM – CALCULATING YOUR BASAL METABOLIC RATE (BMR)

Before we dive into the complexities of macronutrients, let's start with something fundamental to the IIFYM approach: understanding your Basal Metabolic Rate (BMR). BMR is the number of calories your body requires to perform essential functions—like breathing, circulating blood, and regulating body temperature—while at rest. In other words, it's the minimum energy requirement your body needs to survive if you were to do nothing but rest all day.

Calculating your BMR is the first step in determining how many calories—and thus what balance of macros—you need each day. It's a personal number that takes into account your weight, height, age, and gender.

How to Calculate Your BMR

While there are several equations to calculate BMR, one of the most commonly used is the Mifflin-St Jeor Equation:

For men:
BMR = 10 * weight(kg) + 6.25 * height(cm) - 5 * age(y) + 5

For women:
BMR = 10 * weight(kg) + 6.25 * height(cm) - 5 * age(y) - 161

In these equations, weight is in kilograms, height is in centimeters, and age is in years. If you typically use pounds and inches, remember that 1 kilogram equals approximately 2.2 pounds, and 1 inch is equivalent to 2.54 centimeters.

To illustrate, let's calculate the BMR for a 30-year-old woman who is 5'5" (165 cm) and weighs 150 lbs (68 kg):

BMR = [10 * 68kg] + [6.25 * 165cm] - [5 * 30 years] - 161
BMR = 680 + 1031.25 - 150 - 161
BMR = 1400.25

So, her body needs roughly 1400 calories each day to perform essential functions at rest.

BMR and Weight Management

Understanding your BMR is crucial for managing your weight, whether your goal is to lose, gain, or maintain. Here's why:

If you consume fewer calories than your BMR, your body enters a calorie deficit, leading to weight loss as it taps into stored fat for energy. On the other hand, if you consume more than your BMR, your body enters a calorie surplus, which can result in weight gain as excess energy is stored as fat. If your calorie intake is equal to your BMR, your weight will likely stay the same as your intake matches the energy needed for basic functions.

However, remember that BMR is only a part of the equation. It doesn't account for the additional calories you burn through physical activity or the food you eat, known as the thermic effect of food. We'll delve more into these topics in the next chapter when we discuss Total Daily Energy Expenditure (TDEE).

As we navigate the IIFYM journey, it's crucial to

remember that these numbers, while essential for planning, are starting points. They don't consider variables like muscle mass, body composition, or metabolic variations between individuals. Therefore, it's essential to adjust your dietary plans based on progress and individual responses.

Now, armed with an understanding of BMR, you've taken a significant step towards mastering your metabolism. As we move forward, we'll build upon this knowledge, gradually creating a personalized dietary plan that fits not just your macros but your lifestyle too. After all, IIFYM isn't just a diet—it's a lifestyle that empowers you to take control of your nutrition and health.

CHAPTER 3: CALCULATING ENERGY: UNDERSTANDING YOUR TOTAL DAILY ENERGY EXPENDITURE (TDEE)

After understanding and calculating your Basal Metabolic Rate (BMR) in the previous chapter, the next critical step is to calculate your Total Daily Energy Expenditure (TDEE). Your TDEE is a more accurate measure of your total energy needs for the day, encompassing not just your BMR but also the energy expended through physical activity and the thermic effect of food.

What is TDEE?

TDEE is the total number of calories you burn in a day, accounting for all activities: from intense workouts to fidgeting, and even the energy it takes to digest food. It is comprised of three main components:

1. Basal Metabolic Rate (BMR): As discussed in the previous chapter, this is the number of calories your body needs to perform basic life-sustaining functions at rest.

2. Physical Activity Level (PAL): This accounts for the calories burned through all forms of physical activity, such as exercise, walking, chores, and general movement throughout the day.

3. Thermic Effect of Food (TEF): This represents the calories burned through digesting, absorbing, and utilizing the nutrients you consume. It typically accounts for about 10% of your TDEE.

Your TDEE is vital in tailoring your IIFYM diet because it tells you how many calories you need to consume to maintain your current weight given your current level of activity. Depending on your goals (weight loss, weight gain, or maintenance), you can adjust your calorie intake accordingly.

How to Calculate Your TDEE

Calculating your TDEE involves two steps: calculating your BMR (as we've covered in the previous chapter) and then adjusting that number based on your activity level.

Activity levels are typically categorized as follows:

- Sedentary (little or no exercise): BMR * 1.2
- Lightly active (light exercise/sports 1-3 days/week): BMR * 1.375
- Moderately active (moderate exercise/sports 3-5 days/week): BMR * 1.55
- Very active (hard exercise/sports 6-7 days a week): BMR * 1.725
- Extra active (very hard exercise/physical job & exercise 2x/day): BMR * 1.9

To find your TDEE, you multiply your BMR by the factor that best represents your activity level. Let's continue with the example from the previous chapter: a 30-year-old woman who is 5'5" (165 cm), weighs 150 lbs (68 kg), and has a BMR of 1400.25 calories. If she exercises moderately 3-5 days a week, her TDEE would be:

TDEE = BMR * Activity Level
TDEE = 1400.25 * 1.55
TDEE = 2170.39 calories

So, she needs roughly 2170 calories per day to maintain her current weight given her current level of activity.

Applying TDEE to Your Goals

Understanding your TDEE is crucial for setting your calorie and macronutrient goals. If your aim is to lose weight, you'll want to consume fewer calories than your TDEE (creating a calorie deficit). If you want to gain weight, you'll need to consume more (creating a calorie surplus). If you aim to maintain your current weight, you'll aim to consume approximately the same amount of calories as your TDEE.

As you progress through your IIFYM journey, remember that your TDEE is not static. It may change with alterations in your weight, age, or activity level. Consequently, you'll need to recalculate and adjust your macros as needed.

By understanding and applying the concept of TDEE, you've now added a powerful tool to your nutrition toolbox. In the upcoming chapters, we will delve into how to distribute your calories into macronutrients and how to adjust them to fit your unique goals and lifestyle, helping you further customize your IIFYM diet plan. Remember, knowledge is power—and the more you understand about your body and its energy needs, the more successful you'll be in achieving and maintaining your health goals.

CHAPTER 4: TAILORING YOUR MACROS – ALIGNING YOUR NUTRITION WITH YOUR GOALS

With your Basal Metabolic Rate (BMR) and Total Daily Energy Expenditure (TDEE) in hand, you've already won half the battle. Now, it's time to delve into the heart of the IIFYM approach: calculating your macro ratios according to your specific goals. Whether you're seeking to lose weight, gain muscle, or maintain your current weight, aligning your macros with your goals is crucial.

Understanding Macro Ratios

A 'macro ratio' refers to the percentage of your daily

calorie intake that each macronutrient (protein, carbohydrates, and fats) represents. For example, a macro ratio of 40:30:30 means that 40% of your calories come from carbohydrates, 30% from protein, and 30% from fats.

While the exact macro ratio can vary depending on personal preferences and specific dietary goals, a common starting point for many individuals following the IIFYM approach is a 40:30:30 ratio (carbs:protein:fats). This ratio is often suitable for maintaining weight or general health, but if your goal involves weight loss, muscle gain, or other specific outcomes, you may need to tweak the ratio to fit your needs.

Setting Your Macro Ratios According to Your Goals

- **Weight Loss:** If your goal is to lose weight, you may need a higher protein ratio to help preserve lean mass during caloric deficit. A ratio like 30:40:30 (carbs:protein:fats) might be a good starting point.

- **Muscle Gain:** If your goal is muscle gain, you'll likely need more of both protein and carbs to support muscle synthesis and provide sufficient energy for your workouts. In this case, you might aim for something like 40:35:25.

- **Weight Maintenance or General Health**: If you're simply aiming to maintain your current weight or focus on general health, the balanced approach of 40:30:30 often works well.

Calculating Your Macros

Once you have your TDEE and your macro ratios, you can calculate how much of each macronutrient you need in grams. Since each macronutrient provides a specific amount of calories per gram (protein and carbs provide 4 calories per gram, and fats provide 9), you can use these values to convert your calorie goals into gram goals.

For example, if your TDEE is 2170 calories and you're aiming for a 30:40:30 ratio for weight loss, here's how you would calculate your macros:

1. **Carbs:** 30% of 2170 = 651 calories from carbs. Since each gram of carbs provides 4 calories, 651/4 = 162.75 grams of carbs.

2. **Protein:** 40% of 2170 = 868 calories from protein. Since each gram of protein also provides 4 calories, 868/4 = 217 grams of protein.

3. **Fats:** 30% of 2170 = 651 calories from fats. Since each gram of fat provides 9 calories, 651/9 = 72.33 grams of fat.

So, to achieve weight loss, this individual would aim for approximately 163 grams of carbs, 217 grams of protein, and 72 grams of fat each day.

Making Adjustments

Remember that these calculations are only starting points. It's essential to monitor your progress, listen to your body, and adjust your macros as needed. Factors like hunger levels, energy, strength, and changes in weight or body composition can all provide valuable feedback.

As you navigate your IIFYM journey, know that it's more than a diet—it's a flexible approach that allows you to align your nutrition with your lifestyle and goals. Armed with the tools to calculate your BMR, TDEE, and macro ratios, you're now well-equipped to take control of your nutrition and make the IIFYM approach work for you.

IIFYM SNACKS

GREEK YOGURT PARFAIT

Ingredients:
- 1 cup of non-fat Greek yogurt
- 1/2 cup of mixed berries (blueberries, strawberries, raspberries, blackberries)
- 1 tablespoon of honey
- 2 tablespoons of granola
- A sprinkle of chia seeds (optional)

Instructions:

1. Layer half of the Greek yogurt at the bottom of a glass or jar.
2. Add half of the mixed berries on top of the yogurt.
3. Drizzle half of the honey over the berries.
4. Sprinkle 1 tablespoon of granola over the honey.
5. Repeat the process with the remaining ingredients, creating another layer of yogurt, berries, honey, and granola.
6. If desired, sprinkle a small amount of chia seeds on top for some extra fiber and

omega-3 fatty acids.

7. Enjoy immediately or refrigerate for up to 2 hours before eating.

Macronutrient Breakdown:

- Greek yogurt is high in protein, low in fat, and contains some carbs.
- Mixed berries are a great source of fiber and have a small amount of protein and carbs.
- Honey provides mainly carbs.
- Granola is usually high in carbs and contains moderate amounts of protein and fat, depending on the brand and variety.
- Chia seeds are a great source of omega-3 fatty acids, fiber, and also have some protein.

This recipe is a great example of IIFYM because it contains a balance of all three macronutrients, and the quantities can be adjusted to fit your specific macronutrient goals. Just remember to measure and record your food to ensure accuracy in tracking your macros.

PROTEIN-PACKED PEANUT BUTTER BANANA SMOOTHIE

Ingredients:
- 1 medium banana
- 1 cup of unsweetened almond milk
- 1 scoop of protein powder (vanilla or chocolate)
- 2 tablespoons of natural peanut butter
- 1/2 cup of ice
- 1 tablespoon of flax seeds (optional)

Instructions:
1. Peel the banana and cut it into chunks.
2. Add the banana chunks, almond milk, protein powder, peanut butter, and ice to a blender.
3. Blend until smooth and creamy.
4. If desired, add flax seeds and blend for a few more seconds until they're well-

incorporated.
5. Pour the smoothie into a glass and enjoy immediately.

Macronutrient Breakdown:
- Banana provides carbohydrates and a small amount of protein.
- Almond milk is low in carbs, protein, and fat.
- Protein powder is high in protein and can contain carbs and fats, depending on the brand and variety.
- Peanut butter is high in healthy fats and also provides a good amount of protein and a small number of carbs.
- Flax seeds are a great source of omega-3 fatty acids, fiber, and also provide some protein.

Remember to adjust the quantities to fit your personal macronutrient targets. Enjoy your healthy and macro-friendly snack!

AVOCADO EGG SALAD

Ingredients:
- 2 hard-boiled eggs
- 1 ripe avocado
- 1 tablespoon of Greek yogurt
- 1 teaspoon of Dijon mustard
- Salt and pepper to taste
- A handful of cherry tomatoes
- Whole grain bread (optional)

Instructions:
1. Peel the hard-boiled eggs and chop them into small pieces.
2. Cut the avocado in half, remove the pit, and scoop out the flesh.
3. In a bowl, mash the avocado until it's relatively smooth.
4. Add the chopped eggs, Greek yogurt, Dijon mustard, salt, and pepper to the bowl.
5. Mix everything together until well combined.
6. Serve the avocado egg salad with cherry tomatoes on the side for some extra

freshness. If you're looking for some extra carbs, you can serve it on a slice of whole grain bread.

Macronutrient Breakdown:
- Eggs are a great source of protein and healthy fats.
- Avocado is high in healthy monounsaturated fats and contains some protein and fiber.
- Greek yogurt provides protein.
- Dijon mustard is low in all macros but adds flavor.
- Cherry tomatoes and whole grain bread provide carbohydrates.

As always, adjust quantities to fit your specific macronutrient needs. This is a versatile and nutritious snack that can be made in advance, making it great for those busy days when you still want to stick to your macro goals. Enjoy!

CHICKPEA SALAD

Ingredients:

- 1 cup of canned chickpeas, drained and rinsed
- 1 medium cucumber, diced
- 1 medium tomato, diced
- 1/4 of a red onion, finely diced
- 1 tablespoon of olive oil
- 1 tablespoon of lemon juice
- Salt and pepper to taste
- A handful of fresh parsley, chopped (optional)

Instructions:

1. In a bowl, combine the chickpeas, cucumber, tomato, and red onion.
2. In a separate smaller bowl, whisk together the olive oil, lemon juice, salt, and pepper to create a dressing.
3. Pour the dressing over the chickpea mixture and toss everything to combine.
4. If desired, sprinkle chopped parsley over the salad for added flavor and color.
5. Let the salad sit for a few minutes to allow the flavors to blend together, then serve.

Macronutrient Breakdown:

- Chickpeas are a great source of protein and

fiber and contain some healthy carbs.

- Cucumber, tomato, and red onion are high in fiber and have a small amount of carbs.
- Olive oil is a great source of healthy fats.
- Lemon juice provides a small number of carbs.

You can adjust the amount of each ingredient to suit your personal macro goals. This salad is a versatile dish that you can enjoy on its own or as a side dish. Enjoy your healthy, macro-friendly snack!

MIXED BERRY PROTEIN SMOOTHIE BOWL

Ingredients:

- 1 scoop of protein powder (vanilla or unflavored)
- 1 cup of frozen mixed berries
- 1/2 cup of unsweetened almond milk
- Toppings: 1 tablespoon of almond butter, a sprinkle of granola, a few slices of fresh banana or strawberries, a sprinkle of chia seeds

Instructions:

1. Add the protein powder, frozen berries, and almond milk to a blender.
2. Blend until it reaches a thick, ice-cream-like consistency. You might need to stop and stir a couple of times to help it along.
3. Pour the smoothie into a bowl.
4. Drizzle the almond butter over the smoothie.
5. Sprinkle the granola and fresh fruit over the top.

6. Finish with a sprinkle of chia seeds.
7. Enjoy with a spoon, savoring it like a delicious, frosty dessert.

Macronutrient Breakdown:
- Protein powder is high in protein, with varying amounts of carbs and fat depending on the brand.
- Mixed berries provide fiber and carbs, with a small amount of protein.
- Almond milk is low in carbs, protein, and fat.
- Almond butter provides healthy fats, protein, and a small amount of carbs.
- Granola is high in carbs, with moderate protein and fat, depending on the brand.
- Bananas and strawberries provide additional carbs, fiber, and a small amount of protein.
- Chia seeds are a great source of fiber, omega-3 fatty acids, and protein.

As with all recipes, you can adjust the ingredient quantities and choice of toppings to fit your specific macronutrient needs. This recipe is a delicious and satisfying way to enjoy a protein-packed meal or snack that feels like a treat.

HIGH-PROTEIN TUNA SALAD WRAP

Ingredients:

- 1 can of tuna in water, drained
- 2 tablespoons of Greek yogurt
- 1/4 of a red onion, finely diced
- 1/2 of a celery stalk, finely diced
- 1 small apple, diced
- Salt and pepper to taste
- 1 large whole wheat wrap or tortilla
- A handful of spinach or lettuce

Instructions:

1. In a bowl, mix the drained tuna, Greek yogurt, red onion, celery, and apple.
2. Add salt and pepper to taste and stir until well combined.
3. Lay out the whole wheat wrap and spread the tuna salad evenly over it, leaving a bit of space around the edges.
4. Add the spinach or lettuce on top of the tuna salad.

5. Carefully roll up the wrap, tucking in the edges as you go.
6. Cut the wrap in half if desired, and enjoy immediately.

Macronutrient Breakdown:
- Tuna is a great source of protein.
- Greek yogurt provides additional protein.
- Red onion, celery, and apple provide some carbs and fiber.
- The whole wheat wrap is a source of complex carbs and fiber, with a small amount of protein.
- Spinach or lettuce provides fiber and a few additional nutrients with minimal impact on macros.

You can adjust the ingredient quantities to fit your personal macronutrient needs. For example, you can increase the protein by adding more tuna or Greek yogurt, or increase the carbs by choosing a larger wrap or adding more apple. Enjoy this healthy, satisfying, and macro-friendly snack!

ALMOND JOY PROTEIN BALLS

Ingredients:
- 1 cup of rolled oats
- 1/2 cup of chocolate protein powder
- 1/2 cup of unsweetened shredded coconut
- 1/4 cup of chopped almonds
- 1/4 cup of honey or maple syrup
- 1/4 cup of unsweetened almond milk

Instructions:
1. Combine the oats, protein powder, shredded coconut, and chopped almonds in a large bowl.
2. Add the honey (or maple syrup) and almond milk to the bowl.
3. Mix the ingredients together until everything is evenly distributed and the mixture starts to stick together. If the mixture is too dry, add a bit more almond milk. If it's too wet, add a bit more oats or protein powder.
4. Use your hands to shape the mixture into small balls, about 1 inch in diameter.

5. Place the balls on a plate or baking sheet lined with parchment paper.
6. Refrigerate the protein balls for at least 1 hour to allow them to firm up. They can then be stored in an airtight container in the refrigerator for up to a week.

Macronutrient Breakdown:
- Rolled oats provide complex carbs and a good amount of fiber.
- Protein powder, as the name suggests, is high in protein.
- Shredded coconut and almonds provide healthy fats, fiber, and a small amount of protein.
- Honey or maple syrup adds carbs in the form of sugars.
- Almond milk is low in carbs, protein, and fat.

As always, adjust the quantities to fit your personal macronutrient needs. These protein balls are a delicious, convenient snack that can be enjoyed on the go!

QUINOA AND BLACK BEAN SALAD

Ingredients:

- 1 cup of cooked quinoa
- 1 cup of canned black beans, drained and rinsed
- 1 medium tomato, diced
- 1/2 bell pepper, diced (any color)
- 1/4 red onion, diced
- 1/4 cup of chopped fresh cilantro
- 1 tablespoon of olive oil
- Juice of 1 lime
- Salt and pepper to taste

Instructions:

1. In a large bowl, mix together the quinoa, black beans, tomato, bell pepper, and red onion.
2. In a separate bowl, whisk together the olive oil, lime juice, salt, and pepper to make the dressing.
3. Pour the dressing over the quinoa mixture

and stir until everything is evenly coated.

4. Stir in the chopped cilantro.
5. The salad can be served immediately, but it's best if you can let it sit for a few minutes to let the flavors meld together.

Macronutrient Breakdown:
- Quinoa is a great source of protein and carbs, and also provides some healthy fats.
- Black beans are high in protein and fiber, and also contain some carbs.
- Tomato, bell pepper, and red onion provide fiber and a small amount of carbs.
- Olive oil provides healthy fats.
- Cilantro, lime juice, salt, and pepper add flavor with minimal impact on macros.

You can adjust the ingredient quantities to fit your personal macronutrient needs. This salad is filling and nutritious, making it a great snack or meal for those following an IIFYM diet. Enjoy!

TURKEY LETTUCE WRAPS

Ingredients:
- 1 lb ground turkey
- 1 tablespoon olive oil
- 1 small onion, diced
- 2 cloves of garlic, minced
- 1 bell pepper, diced (any color)
- 1/2 cup of canned water chestnuts, drained and chopped
- 2 tablespoons of low-sodium soy sauce or tamari
- 1 head of iceberg or butter lettuce, leaves separated

Instructions:
1. Heat the olive oil in a large skillet over medium heat.
2. Add the ground turkey and cook until it's no longer pink, breaking it up into small pieces as it cooks.
3. Add the diced onion, minced garlic, and diced bell pepper to the skillet and cook until the vegetables are softened.

4. Stir in the chopped water chestnuts and soy sauce, cooking for another 2-3 minutes until everything is heated through.
5. To serve, spoon some of the turkey mixture into a lettuce leaf and fold it up like a wrap.

Macronutrient Breakdown:
- Ground turkey is a great source of lean protein.
- Olive oil provides healthy fats.
- Onion, garlic, bell pepper, and water chestnuts provide some carbs and fiber.
- Soy sauce adds flavor with minimal impact on macros.
- Lettuce is low in macros but provides volume and crunch to the wrap.

As always, adjust the ingredient quantities to fit your personal macronutrient needs. This is a light, healthy, and satisfying dish that can be enjoyed as a snack or a meal. Enjoy your turkey lettuce wraps!

COTTAGE CHEESE AND PINEAPPLE BOWL

Ingredients:
- 1 cup of low-fat cottage cheese
- 1/2 cup of fresh pineapple, diced
- A sprinkle of cinnamon (optional)
- A few chopped almonds or walnuts (optional)

Instructions:
1. Spoon the cottage cheese into a bowl.
2. Top with the diced pineapple.
3. If desired, sprinkle a bit of cinnamon over the top for extra flavor.
4. If you want to add some healthy fats, sprinkle a few chopped almonds or walnuts over the top.
5. Enjoy immediately.

Macronutrient Breakdown:
- Cottage cheese is a good source of protein, with a small amount of carbs and fat.
- Pineapple provides carbs and fiber, with a small

amount of protein.

- Cinnamon adds flavor with minimal impact on macros.
- Almonds or walnuts provide healthy fats, along with some protein and carbs.

You can adjust the amount of each ingredient to fit your personal macronutrient needs. This bowl is a refreshing and satisfying snack that provides a good balance of macros. Enjoy!

ROASTED CHICKPEAS

Ingredients:

- 1 can (15 ounces) chickpeas, drained and rinsed
- 1 tablespoon of olive oil
- 1/2 teaspoon of smoked paprika
- 1/4 teaspoon of garlic powder
- Salt and pepper to taste

Instructions:

1. Preheat your oven to 400°F (200°C).
2. After rinsing the chickpeas, spread them out on a clean kitchen towel and pat them dry. Removing the moisture helps them get crispier.
3. Toss the chickpeas in a bowl with the olive oil, smoked paprika, garlic powder, salt, and pepper.
4. Spread the chickpeas out in a single layer on a baking sheet.
5. Bake for 20-30 minutes, or until the chickpeas are golden and crispy. Make sure to shake the pan or stir the chickpeas every

10 minutes or so to ensure they roast evenly.

6. Let them cool before eating. They will become crunchier as they cool.

Macronutrient Breakdown:

- Chickpeas are a great source of plant-based protein and fiber, and they also provide some carbs.
- Olive oil is a source of healthy fats.
- Smoked paprika, garlic powder, salt, and pepper add flavor with minimal impact on macros.

This snack can be customized with different spices to fit your preferences. The quantities can also be adjusted to match your personal macronutrient needs. Roasted chickpeas are a healthy, satisfying snack that's easy to make and full of flavor. Enjoy!

PEANUT BUTTER PROTEIN BARS

Ingredients:
- 2 cups of rolled oats
- 1 cup of protein powder (vanilla or unflavored)
- 1/2 cup of natural peanut butter
- 1/4 cup of honey or maple syrup
- 1/2 cup of unsweetened almond milk
- Optional: a handful of dark chocolate chips for topping

Instructions:
1. In a large bowl, combine the rolled oats and protein powder.
2. In a microwave-safe bowl, combine the peanut butter and honey. Microwave for about 20-30 seconds until they're easier to mix together.
3. Pour the peanut butter mixture into the bowl with the oats and protein powder. Stir until the dry ingredients are coated.
4. Gradually add the almond milk, stirring until a thick dough forms. You want the mixture to be moist, but not too wet.

5. Press the mixture into a baking dish lined with parchment paper.
6. If using, sprinkle the chocolate chips on top and press them gently into the mixture.
7. Refrigerate for at least 2 hours, or until the bars are firm.
8. Cut into bars and store in an airtight container in the refrigerator.

Macronutrient Breakdown:
- Rolled oats provide complex carbs and fiber.
- Protein powder is high in protein.
- Peanut butter provides healthy fats and some protein.
- Honey or maple syrup adds some carbs in the form of sugars.
- Almond milk is low in macros but helps to bind everything together.
- Dark chocolate chips add a bit of sugar, fat, and a touch of protein.

Remember, you can adjust the quantities to fit your personal macronutrient needs. These bars are a convenient, satisfying snack that you can enjoy on the go. Enjoy!

NO-BAKE CHOCOLATE PROTEIN BALLS

Ingredients:
- 1 cup of rolled oats
- 1 cup of chocolate protein powder
- 1/2 cup of natural almond butter
- 1/4 cup of honey or maple syrup
- 1/3 cup of unsweetened almond milk
- Optional: a handful of mini dark chocolate chips

Instructions:
1. In a large bowl, combine the rolled oats and protein powder.
2. In a microwave-safe bowl, combine the almond butter and honey. Microwave for about 20-30 seconds until they're easier to mix together.
3. Pour the almond butter mixture into the bowl with the oats and protein powder. Stir until the dry ingredients are coated.
4. Gradually add the almond milk, stirring

until a thick dough forms. You want the mixture to be moist, but not too wet.

5. Use your hands to shape the dough into balls, each about 1 inch in diameter.
6. If using, press a few mini chocolate chips into each ball.
7. Place the protein balls on a tray or plate lined with parchment paper and refrigerate for at least 1 hour to allow them to firm up.
8. Store in an airtight container in the refrigerator.

Macronutrient Breakdown:
- Rolled oats provide complex carbs and fiber.
- Chocolate protein powder is high in protein and gives the balls a chocolatey flavor.
- Almond butter provides healthy fats and a bit of protein.
- Honey or maple syrup adds a bit of sweetness and carbs.
- Almond milk is low in macros but helps to bind everything together.
- Dark chocolate chips add a bit of sugar, fat, and a touch of protein.

Remember to adjust the quantities to suit your personal macronutrient needs. These protein balls are a delicious, satisfying snack that you can enjoy on the go. Enjoy!

HUMMUS AND VEGGIE WRAP

Ingredients:
- 1 large whole wheat tortilla or wrap
- 2 tablespoons of hummus
- A handful of spinach or lettuce
- 1 small carrot, grated
- 1/2 bell pepper, thinly sliced (any color)
- 1/4 of a cucumber, thinly sliced
- A few slices of avocado

Instructions:
1. Spread the hummus evenly over the whole wheat wrap.
2. Lay out the spinach or lettuce on top of the hummus.
3. Add the grated carrot, sliced bell pepper, and sliced cucumber on top of the greens.
4. Arrange the avocado slices on top of the other vegetables.
5. Roll up the wrap carefully, tucking in the sides as you go.
6. Cut in half and enjoy immediately, or wrap in foil for a portable snack.

Macronutrient Breakdown:
- Whole wheat wrap provides complex carbs and some protein.
- Hummus provides healthy fats and a bit of protein.
- Spinach or lettuce, carrot, bell pepper, and cucumber provide fiber and a small amount of carbs.
- Avocado provides healthy fats, fiber, and a small amount of protein.

Remember, you can adjust the quantities and selection of vegetables to fit your personal macronutrient needs. This wrap is a fresh, nutritious, and satisfying snack that's perfect for those following an IIFYM diet. Enjoy!

BANANA ALMOND SMOOTHIE

Ingredients:

- 1 medium banana
- 1 cup of unsweetened almond milk
- 1 tablespoon of almond butter or peanut butter
- 1 scoop of vanilla protein powder
- 1/4 cup of raw, unsalted almonds or walnuts
- Ice cubes

Instructions:

1. In a blender, add the banana, almond milk, almond or peanut butter, protein powder, and nuts.
2. Blend until the mixture is smooth. If it's too thick, you can add a little more almond milk; if it's too thin, you can add a few more nuts or half a banana.
3. Once the mixture is your desired consistency, add a few ice cubes and blend again until it's chilled.
4. Pour into a glass and enjoy immediately.

Macronutrient Breakdown:

- Banana provides complex carbs and a bit of protein.
- Almond milk is low in macros but provides volume to the smoothie.
- Almond or peanut butter, as well as raw nuts, provide healthy fats and some protein.
- Protein powder is a great source of protein.

Remember, you can adjust the quantities to fit your personal macronutrient needs. This smoothie is a nutritious, satisfying snack that can be enjoyed any time of the day. Enjoy!

BAKED SWEET POTATO WITH GREEK YOGURT

Ingredients:
- 1 medium sweet potato
- 1/2 cup of non-fat Greek yogurt
- A sprinkle of cinnamon (optional)
- A drizzle of honey or pure maple syrup (optional)

Instructions:
1. Preheat your oven to 400°F (200°C).
2. Prick the sweet potato with a fork several times and place it on a baking sheet.
3. Bake for about 45 minutes, or until the sweet potato is cooked through and tender.
4. Let the sweet potato cool for a few minutes, then slice it open lengthwise.
5. Top the sweet potato with the Greek yogurt.
6. If desired, sprinkle a bit of cinnamon over the top and drizzle with honey or maple syrup.
7. Enjoy immediately.

Macronutrient Breakdown:
- Sweet potato is a great source of complex carbs and fiber, and it also contains some protein.
- Non-fat Greek yogurt is high in protein.
- Cinnamon adds flavor with minimal impact on macros.
- Honey or maple syrup adds a bit of sweetness and carbs.

You can adjust the quantities to fit your personal macronutrient needs. This is a filling, nutritious snack that offers a good balance of protein, carbs, and fiber. Enjoy!

TUNA AND AVOCADO STUFFED BELL PEPPERS

Ingredients:
- 2 bell peppers (any color), halved and seeds removed
- 1 can of tuna in water, drained
- 1 ripe avocado, mashed
- 1/4 cup of diced red onion
- 1 tablespoon of fresh lemon juice
- Salt and pepper to taste

Instructions:
1. Preheat your oven to 375°F (190°C).
2. Place the halved bell peppers cut side up on a baking sheet and roast for about 20 minutes, or until they're tender.
3. While the peppers are roasting, mix the tuna, mashed avocado, red onion, and lemon juice in a bowl. Season with salt and

pepper.

4. When the bell peppers are done, remove them from the oven and let them cool slightly.
5. Spoon the tuna mixture into each bell pepper half.
6. Serve immediately, or store in the fridge for later.

Macronutrient Breakdown:
- Bell peppers are low in calories and provide some carbs.
- Tuna is a great source of lean protein.
- Avocado provides healthy fats and fiber.
- Red onion adds some carbs and flavor.
- Lemon juice adds flavor with minimal impact on macros.

Remember, you can adjust the quantities to fit your personal macronutrient needs. This is a nutritious, protein-packed snack that's also very filling. Enjoy your Tuna and Avocado Stuffed Bell Peppers!

APPLE ALMOND BUTTER SANDWICH

Ingredients:
- 1 medium apple
- 2 tablespoons of almond butter
- A sprinkle of granola or chopped nuts (optional)

Instructions:
1. Slice the apple into round, flat discs, about 1/4 inch thick. You'll need two slices for each 'sandwich'.
2. Spread a tablespoon of almond butter onto one side of an apple slice.
3. If using, sprinkle a bit of granola or chopped nuts on top of the almond butter.
4. Place another apple slice on top, creating a 'sandwich'.
5. Repeat with the remaining apple slices and almond butter.
6. Enjoy immediately, or store in an airtight container in the fridge for later.

Macronutrient Breakdown:

- Apple provides healthy carbs and fiber.
- Almond butter is a source of healthy fats and protein.
- Granola or nuts add some complex carbs, healthy fats, and protein.

Remember to adjust the quantities to match your personal macronutrient needs. This Apple Almond Butter Sandwich is a fun and nutritious snack that combines sweet, crisp apples with rich, creamy almond butter. Enjoy!

YOGURT & BERRY PARFAIT

Ingredients:
- 1 cup of non-fat Greek yogurt
- 1/2 cup of mixed berries (such as strawberries, blueberries, and raspberries)
- 1 tablespoon of honey or maple syrup
- 2 tablespoons of granola

Instructions:
1. In a cup or jar, layer half of the Greek yogurt at the bottom.
2. Add a layer of half of the mixed berries on top of the yogurt.
3. Drizzle half of the honey or maple syrup over the berries.
4. Sprinkle half of the granola on top.
5. Repeat the layers with the remaining yogurt, berries, sweetener, and granola.
6. Enjoy immediately, or refrigerate for up to a day before eating.

Macronutrient Breakdown:
- Greek yogurt is high in protein.

- Berries provide healthy carbs and fiber.
- Honey or maple syrup adds a bit of sweetness and carbs.
- Granola provides complex carbs, a bit of protein, and some healthy fats.

You can adjust the quantities to fit your personal macronutrient needs. This Greek Yogurt Berry Parfait is a delicious, nutritious snack that offers a good balance of protein, carbs, and a bit of healthy fat. It's perfect for a breakfast on the go, a post-workout snack, or a healthy dessert. Enjoy!

ROASTED EDAMAME

Ingredients:
- 2 cups of frozen edamame (shelled)
- 1 tablespoon of olive oil
- 1 teaspoon of garlic powder
- 1/2 teaspoon of smoked paprika
- 1/2 teaspoon of sea salt
- Optional: a pinch of cayenne pepper for some heat

Instructions:
1. Preheat your oven to 400°F (200°C).
2. In a bowl, toss the frozen edamame with olive oil, garlic powder, smoked paprika, sea salt, and cayenne pepper (if using). Mix until the edamame is evenly coated with the seasonings.
3. Spread the seasoned edamame on a baking sheet in a single layer.
4. Roast in the oven for 15-20 minutes, or until the edamame is crispy and slightly golden.
5. Remove from the oven and let them cool for

a few minutes before serving.

Macronutrient Breakdown:
- Edamame is a great source of plant-based protein and fiber, and it also contains carbohydrates.
- Olive oil provides healthy fats.
- Garlic powder, smoked paprika, sea salt, and cayenne pepper add flavor with minimal impact on macros.

You can adjust the quantities and seasonings to fit your personal macronutrient needs and taste preferences. These roasted edamame make for a crunchy and protein-rich snack that's perfect for satisfying your cravings. Enjoy!

ZUCCHINI FRITTERS

Ingredients:
- 2 medium zucchinis, grated
- 1/4 cup of almond flour or whole wheat flour
- 2 tablespoons of grated Parmesan cheese (optional)
- 1 large egg, beaten
- 1/4 teaspoon of garlic powder
- 1/4 teaspoon of onion powder
- Salt and pepper to taste
- 1 tablespoon of olive oil (for cooking)

Instructions:
1. Place the grated zucchini in a clean kitchen towel or cheesecloth and squeeze out any excess moisture.
2. In a large bowl, combine the grated zucchini, almond flour (or whole wheat flour), Parmesan cheese (if using), beaten egg, garlic powder, onion powder, salt, and pepper. Mix well until everything is evenly incorporated.
3. Heat olive oil in a skillet over medium heat.

4. Take about 1/4 cup of the zucchini mixture and form it into a patty. Repeat with the remaining mixture.
5. Place the patties in the skillet and cook for 2-3 minutes on each side, or until golden brown.
6. Remove the fritters from the skillet and let them cool slightly before serving.

Macronutrient Breakdown:

- Zucchini is low in carbs and calories, and it provides fiber.
- Almond flour or whole wheat flour adds complex carbs and some protein.
- Parmesan cheese (if using) adds a bit of protein and flavor.
- The egg provides additional protein and helps bind the fritters together.
- Garlic powder, onion powder, salt, and pepper add flavor with minimal impact on macros.
- Olive oil provides healthy fats.

You can adjust the quantities to fit your personal macronutrient needs. These zucchini fritters are a tasty and nutrient-packed snack that can be enjoyed on their own or served with a dip of your choice. Enjoy!

PROTEIN-PACKED EGG MUFFINS

Ingredients:
- 6 large eggs
- 1/4 cup of milk (any type you prefer)
- 1/2 cup of chopped vegetables (such as spinach, bell peppers, onions, or mushrooms)
- 1/4 cup of shredded cheese (optional)
- Salt and pepper to taste

Instructions:
1. Preheat your oven to 350°F (175°C) and grease a muffin tin with cooking spray or oil.
2. In a bowl, whisk together the eggs, milk, salt, and pepper until well combined.
3. Stir in the chopped vegetables and shredded cheese (if using).
4. Pour the egg mixture evenly into the prepared muffin tin, filling each cup about three-quarters full.
5. Bake for 18-20 minutes, or until the egg muffins are set and slightly golden on top.
6. Remove from the oven and let them cool

in the muffin tin for a few minutes before transferring to a wire rack.

7. Enjoy them warm or refrigerate for later consumption.

Macronutrient Breakdown:
- Eggs are a great source of protein and healthy fats.
- Milk adds a small amount of protein and helps make the egg mixture fluffy.
- Chopped vegetables provide fiber and a variety of vitamins and minerals.
- Shredded cheese (if using) adds a bit of protein and flavor.
- Salt and pepper add taste with minimal impact on macros.

You can adjust the quantities and choice of vegetables to fit your personal macronutrient needs and taste preferences. These protein-packed egg muffins are convenient, versatile, and perfect for meal prep or on-the-go snacking. Enjoy!

BAKED KALE CHIPS

Ingredients:
- 1 bunch of kale
- 1 tablespoon of olive oil
- Salt and pepper to taste
- Optional: additional seasonings such as garlic powder, paprika, or nutritional yeast

Instructions:
1. Preheat your oven to 300°F (150°C) and line a baking sheet with parchment paper.
2. Wash and thoroughly dry the kale leaves. Remove the tough stems and tear the leaves into bite-sized pieces.
3. In a large bowl, toss the kale pieces with olive oil, salt, pepper, and any additional seasonings of your choice. Make sure the leaves are evenly coated.
4. Spread the seasoned kale leaves out in a single layer on the prepared baking sheet.
5. Bake for 10-15 minutes, or until the kale chips are crisp and slightly browned. Keep a close eye on them to prevent burning.

6. Remove from the oven and let the chips cool on the baking sheet for a few minutes before transferring to a wire rack to cool completely.

Macronutrient Breakdown:
- Kale is low in calories and carbs, and it provides fiber.
- Olive oil adds healthy fats.
- Salt, pepper, and optional seasonings add flavor with minimal impact on macros.

You can adjust the quantities and seasonings to fit your personal macronutrient needs and taste preferences. These baked kale chips are a nutritious and satisfying alternative to traditional potato chips. Enjoy the crispy, flavorful snack guilt-free!

CUCUMBER SUSHI ROLLS

Ingredients:
- 1 large cucumber
- 4-6 slices of cooked chicken breast or deli turkey
- 1/4 avocado, sliced
- 2 tablespoons of low-sodium soy sauce or tamari
- 1 tablespoon of rice vinegar
- Optional: sesame seeds for garnish

Instructions:
1. Peel the cucumber and cut it lengthwise into thin strips using a vegetable peeler or mandoline slicer.
2. Lay out one cucumber strip and place a slice of chicken breast or turkey and a few slices of avocado along one end.
3. Gently roll up the cucumber strip, starting from the end with the fillings, to form a sushi-like roll.
4. Repeat the process with the remaining cucumber strips, chicken breast or turkey,

and avocado.

5. In a small bowl, mix the low-sodium soy sauce or tamari with the rice vinegar to make a dipping sauce.

6. Sprinkle sesame seeds on top of the rolls for garnish, if desired.

7. Serve the cucumber sushi rolls with the dipping sauce on the side.

Macronutrient Breakdown:

- Cucumber is low in calories and provides hydration.
- Cooked chicken breast or deli turkey is a lean source of protein.
- Avocado adds healthy fats and some fiber.
- Low-sodium soy sauce or tamari provides a savory flavor.
- Rice vinegar adds a tangy taste.

You can adjust the quantities and choice of fillings to fit your personal macronutrient needs and taste preferences. These cucumber sushi rolls offer a refreshing and nutritious twist on traditional sushi. Enjoy the light and satisfying snack!

PROTEIN-PACKED CHOCOLATE CHIA PUDDING

Ingredients:

- 2 tablespoons of chia seeds
- 1 cup of unsweetened almond milk (or any milk of your choice)
- 1 scoop of chocolate protein powder
- 1 tablespoon of unsweetened cocoa powder
- 1 tablespoon of honey or maple syrup (optional, for added sweetness)
- Optional toppings: sliced strawberries, chopped nuts, or a sprinkle of coconut flakes

Instructions:

1. In a bowl or jar, mix together the chia seeds, almond milk, chocolate protein powder, cocoa powder, and honey or maple syrup (if using). Stir well to combine.
2. Let the mixture sit for a few minutes, then give it another stir to prevent clumping.
3. Cover the bowl or jar and refrigerate for at least 2 hours or overnight, allowing the

chia seeds to absorb the liquid and form a pudding-like consistency.

4. Once the pudding has set, give it a final stir. If it seems too thick, you can add a splash of almond milk to achieve the desired consistency.
5. Serve the chocolate chia pudding in a bowl or glass, and top it with your preferred toppings such as sliced strawberries, chopped nuts, or coconut flakes.

Macronutrient Breakdown:
- Chia seeds provide fiber, healthy fats, and a small amount of protein.
- Almond milk adds moisture and a creamy texture.
- Chocolate protein powder offers additional protein.
- Unsweetened cocoa powder adds a rich chocolate flavor with minimal impact on macros.
- Honey or maple syrup (if using) provides a touch of sweetness.

You can adjust the quantities and sweetness level to fit your personal macronutrient needs and taste preferences. This protein-packed chocolate chia pudding is a satisfying and nutrient-dense snack that will keep you fueled throughout the day. Enjoy!

SWEET POTATO TOAST WITH ALMOND BUTTER AND BANANA

Ingredients:

- 1 medium sweet potato
- 2 tablespoons of almond butter
- 1 small banana, sliced
- Optional toppings: sprinkle of cinnamon, drizzle of honey or maple syrup, or chopped nuts

Instructions:

1. Preheat your oven to 400°F (200°C).
2. Wash the sweet potato and slice it lengthwise into 1/4-inch thick slices.
3. Place the sweet potato slices on a baking sheet lined with parchment paper.
4. Bake for about 15-20 minutes, or until the sweet potato slices are tender and slightly golden.

5. Let the sweet potato slices cool for a few minutes.
6. Spread a thin layer of almond butter on each sweet potato slice.
7. Arrange the banana slices on top of the almond butter.
8. If desired, sprinkle cinnamon, drizzle honey or maple syrup, or sprinkle chopped nuts over the toppings.
9. Enjoy immediately.

Macronutrient Breakdown:

- Sweet potato provides complex carbs, fiber, and some vitamins.
- Almond butter adds healthy fats and a bit of protein.
- Banana offers natural sugars, potassium, and additional fiber.
- Optional toppings provide additional flavor and nutrients.

You can adjust the quantities and toppings to fit your personal macronutrient needs and taste preferences. This Sweet Potato Toast with Almond Butter and Banana is a delicious and nutritious snack that offers a satisfying combination of sweet and creamy flavors. Enjoy!

PROTEIN-PACKED ENERGY BALLS

Ingredients:
- 1 cup of rolled oats
- 1/2 cup of almond butter or peanut butter
- 1/4 cup of honey or maple syrup
- 1/4 cup of protein powder (vanilla or chocolate)
- 2 tablespoons of chia seeds
- 2 tablespoons of mini chocolate chips or chopped nuts (optional)
- 1/2 teaspoon of vanilla extract
- Pinch of salt

Instructions:
1. In a large bowl, combine the rolled oats, almond butter or peanut butter, honey or maple syrup, protein powder, chia seeds, mini chocolate chips or chopped nuts (if using), vanilla extract, and salt.
2. Stir until all the ingredients are well mixed and form a sticky dough.
3. Using your hands, roll the dough into small balls, about 1 inch in diameter.

4. Place the energy balls on a baking sheet lined with parchment paper.
5. Refrigerate the energy balls for at least 30 minutes, or until firm.
6. Once chilled, transfer the energy balls to an airtight container and store in the refrigerator.

Macronutrient Breakdown:
- Rolled oats provide complex carbs and fiber.
- Almond butter or peanut butter offers healthy fats and some protein.
- Honey or maple syrup adds a touch of sweetness and carbs.
- Protein powder boosts the protein content.
- Chia seeds provide additional fiber and healthy fats.
- Mini chocolate chips or chopped nuts (if using) add a bit of flavor and texture.

You can adjust the quantities and optional ingredients to fit your personal macronutrient needs and taste preferences. These protein-packed energy balls are a convenient and delicious snack to satisfy your hunger and provide a boost of energy throughout the day. Enjoy!

CAPRESE SKEWERS

Ingredients:

- Cherry or grape tomatoes
- Fresh mozzarella cheese, cut into bite-sized pieces
- Fresh basil leaves
- Balsamic glaze or balsamic reduction
- Skewers or toothpicks

Instructions:

1. Wash the cherry or grape tomatoes and pat them dry.
2. On each skewer or toothpick, thread one tomato, followed by a piece of mozzarella cheese, and then a fresh basil leaf.
3. Repeat the process until you have the desired number of skewers.
4. Arrange the Caprese skewers on a serving platter.
5. Drizzle balsamic glaze or balsamic reduction over the skewers.
6. Serve immediately.

Macronutrient Breakdown:
- Cherry or grape tomatoes provide vitamins, minerals, and fiber.
- Fresh mozzarella cheese offers protein and some healthy fats.
- Fresh basil leaves add flavor and antioxidants.
- Balsamic glaze or balsamic reduction adds a tangy sweetness with minimal impact on macros.

You can adjust the quantities to fit your personal macronutrient needs and taste preferences. These Caprese Skewers are a refreshing and elegant snack that combines the classic flavors of tomatoes, mozzarella, and basil. They're perfect for parties or as a light appetizer. Enjoy!

QUINOA STUFFED BELL PEPPERS

Ingredients:

- 2 large bell peppers (any color), halved and seeds removed
- 1 cup of cooked quinoa
- 1/2 cup of canned black beans, drained and rinsed
- 1/2 cup of corn kernels (fresh or frozen)
- 1/4 cup of diced red onion
- 1/4 cup of diced tomatoes
- 1/4 cup of chopped fresh cilantro
- Juice of 1 lime
- 1 teaspoon of ground cumin
- Salt and pepper to taste
- Optional toppings: shredded cheese, avocado slices, Greek yogurt or sour cream

Instructions:

1. Preheat your oven to 375°F (190°C).
2. Place the bell pepper halves in a baking dish.
3. In a large bowl, combine the cooked quinoa, black beans, corn kernels, red onion, tomatoes, cilantro, lime juice, cumin,

salt, and pepper. Mix well until all the ingredients are evenly incorporated.

4. Spoon the quinoa mixture into each bell pepper half, pressing it down slightly to fill them.
5. Cover the baking dish with foil and bake for about 25-30 minutes, or until the bell peppers are tender and the filling is heated through.
6. Remove the foil and, if desired, sprinkle shredded cheese on top of each stuffed pepper. Return to the oven and bake for an additional 5 minutes, or until the cheese is melted and bubbly.
7. Remove from the oven and let them cool for a few minutes.
8. Serve the quinoa stuffed bell peppers with optional toppings such as avocado slices, Greek yogurt, or sour cream.

Macronutrient Breakdown:
- Bell peppers are low in calories and provide carbs, fiber, and vitamins.
- Quinoa offers complex carbs, protein, and fiber.
- Black beans provide plant-based protein and fiber.
- Corn kernels add carbs and some fiber.
- Red onion, tomatoes, cilantro, lime juice, cumin, salt, and pepper add flavor with minimal impact on macros.
- Optional toppings contribute healthy fats,

additional protein, and creamy textures.

You can adjust the quantities and toppings to fit your personal macronutrient needs and taste preferences. These quinoa stuffed bell peppers are a satisfying and nutritious snack or light meal that's packed with colorful vegetables and wholesome ingredients. Enjoy!

GREEK YOGURT PARFAIT WITH MIXED BERRIES

Ingredients:
- 1 cup of non-fat Greek yogurt
- 1/2 cup of mixed berries (such as strawberries, blueberries, and raspberries)
- 2 tablespoons of granola or crushed nuts
- Optional: drizzle of honey or maple syrup

Instructions:
1. In a glass or bowl, layer half of the Greek yogurt at the bottom.
2. Add a layer of half of the mixed berries on top of the yogurt.
3. Sprinkle a tablespoon of granola or crushed nuts over the berries.
4. Repeat the layers with the remaining yogurt, berries, and granola or crushed nuts.
5. If desired, drizzle a bit of honey or maple syrup over the top.
6. Enjoy immediately.

Macronutrient Breakdown:
- Greek yogurt is high in protein.
- Mixed berries provide vitamins, minerals, and fiber.
- Granola or crushed nuts add complex carbs, healthy fats, and some protein.
- Optional honey or maple syrup provides a touch of sweetness and carbs.

You can adjust the quantities and toppings to fit your personal macronutrient needs and taste preferences. This Greek Yogurt Parfait with Mixed Berries is a refreshing and nutritious snack that offers a balance of protein, carbs, and fiber. It's perfect for a quick breakfast, post-workout snack, or a satisfying dessert. Enjoy!

BAKED GARLIC PARMESAN ZUCCHINI CHIPS

Ingredients:

- 2 medium zucchinis, thinly sliced
- 1/2 cup of grated Parmesan cheese
- 1/2 teaspoon of garlic powder
- 1/4 teaspoon of paprika
- Salt and pepper to taste
- Cooking spray or olive oil

Instructions:

1. Preheat your oven to 425°F (220°C) and line a baking sheet with parchment paper.
2. In a bowl, combine the grated Parmesan cheese, garlic powder, paprika, salt, and pepper.
3. Lightly spray the zucchini slices with cooking spray or toss them in a small amount of olive oil to help the seasoning stick.
4. Dip each zucchini slice into the Parmesan mixture, pressing gently to ensure the

coating sticks to both sides.

5. Place the coated zucchini slices in a single layer on the prepared baking sheet.
6. Bake for about 15-20 minutes, or until the zucchini chips are golden and crispy.
7. Remove from the oven and let them cool on a wire rack for a few minutes to become even crispier.

Macronutrient Breakdown:
- Zucchini is low in calories and provides vitamins, minerals, and fiber.
- Parmesan cheese adds flavor, protein, and a small amount of healthy fats.
- Garlic powder and paprika add savory flavor with minimal impact on macros.
- Salt and pepper enhance taste with minimal macros.

You can adjust the quantities and seasonings to fit your personal macronutrient needs and taste preferences. These Baked Garlic Parmesan Zucchini Chips are a healthier alternative to traditional potato chips. They offer a satisfying crunch and are packed with flavor. Enjoy them as a guilt-free snack or side dish!

APPLE CINNAMON PROTEIN MUFFINS

Ingredients:

- 1 cup of oat flour (you can make your own by blending rolled oats)
- 1/2 cup of vanilla protein powder
- 1 teaspoon of baking powder
- 1/2 teaspoon of ground cinnamon
- 1/4 teaspoon of salt
- 2 large eggs
- 1/4 cup of unsweetened applesauce
- 1/4 cup of almond milk (or any milk of your choice)
- 1 tablespoon of honey or maple syrup
- 1 teaspoon of vanilla extract
- 1 medium apple, peeled and finely chopped

Instructions:

1. Preheat your oven to 350°F (175°C) and line

a muffin tin with paper liners or grease it lightly.

2. In a bowl, whisk together the oat flour, protein powder, baking powder, ground cinnamon, and salt.
3. In a separate bowl, beat the eggs, then add the applesauce, almond milk, honey or maple syrup, and vanilla extract. Mix well to combine.
4. Gradually add the dry ingredients to the wet ingredients, stirring until just combined.
5. Gently fold in the chopped apple.
6. Spoon the batter evenly into the prepared muffin tin, filling each cup about three-quarters full.
7. Bake for 15-18 minutes, or until a toothpick inserted into the center of a muffin comes out clean.
8. Remove from the oven and let the muffins cool in the tin for a few minutes before transferring them to a wire rack to cool completely.

Macronutrient Breakdown:
- Oat flour provides complex carbs and fiber.
- Vanilla protein powder adds protein and flavor.
- Eggs offer additional protein and healthy fats.
- Unsweetened applesauce adds moisture and natural sweetness.
- Almond milk contributes to the moisture and

texture.
- Honey or maple syrup provides sweetness and carbs.
- Chopped apple adds natural sweetness and fiber.

You can adjust the quantities and sweetness level to fit your personal macronutrient needs and taste preferences. These Apple Cinnamon Protein Muffins are a delicious and nutritious snack that's packed with protein and fiber. Enjoy them as a quick grab-and-go option or a satisfying treat!

TURKEY AND HUMMUS ROLL-UPS

Ingredients:

- 4-6 slices of deli turkey
- 4-6 teaspoons of hummus (any flavor you prefer)
- 1/2 cucumber, sliced into thin strips
- 1/2 bell pepper (any color), sliced into thin strips
- 1/4 red onion, thinly sliced
- Optional: lettuce or spinach leaves

Instructions:

1. Lay out one slice of deli turkey on a clean surface.
2. Spread a teaspoon of hummus evenly over the turkey slice.
3. Place a few cucumber strips, bell pepper strips, red onion slices, and optional lettuce or spinach leaves on top of the hummus.
4. Gently roll up the turkey slice, starting from one end, to form a tight roll-up.

5. Repeat the process with the remaining turkey slices and ingredients.
6. Secure each roll-up with a toothpick if needed.
7. Serve the turkey and hummus roll-ups immediately or refrigerate them for later.

Macronutrient Breakdown:
- Deli turkey provides lean protein.
- Hummus offers plant-based protein, healthy fats, and fiber.
- Cucumber, bell pepper, and red onion provide vitamins, minerals, and fiber.
- Lettuce or spinach leaves add additional vitamins and minerals.

You can adjust the quantities and choice of vegetables to fit your personal macronutrient needs and taste preferences. These Turkey and Hummus Roll-Ups are a protein-packed and flavorful snack that's perfect for satisfying your hunger between meals. Enjoy them as a light lunch option or an on-the-go snack!

SPINACH AND FETA STUFFED MUSHROOMS

Ingredients:
- 8 large button or cremini mushrooms
- 1 cup of fresh spinach, finely chopped
- 1/4 cup of crumbled feta cheese
- 2 tablespoons of grated Parmesan cheese
- 2 cloves of garlic, minced
- 1 tablespoon of olive oil
- Salt and pepper to taste

Instructions:
1. Preheat your oven to 375°F (190°C) and line a baking sheet with parchment paper.
2. Remove the stems from the mushrooms and set aside. Place the mushroom caps on the prepared baking sheet, rounded side down.
3. Finely chop the mushroom stems and set aside.
4. In a skillet, heat the olive oil over medium heat. Add the minced garlic and chopped

mushroom stems. Sauté for a few minutes until the mushrooms release their moisture and become tender.

5. Add the chopped spinach to the skillet and cook until wilted. Season with salt and pepper to taste.

6. Remove the skillet from heat and let the mixture cool slightly.

7. In a bowl, combine the sautéed spinach and mushroom mixture with the crumbled feta cheese and grated Parmesan cheese. Stir until well combined.

8. Spoon the spinach and feta mixture into each mushroom cap, pressing it down gently.

9. Bake for approximately 15-20 minutes, or until the mushrooms are tender and the cheese is golden and bubbly.

10. Remove from the oven and let the stuffed mushrooms cool for a few minutes before serving.

Macronutrient Breakdown:

- Mushrooms provide low calories and carbs, along with vitamins and minerals.
- Spinach offers vitamins, minerals, and fiber.
- Feta cheese and Parmesan cheese contribute protein and flavor.
- Olive oil adds healthy fats.

You can adjust the quantities and seasonings to fit your personal macronutrient needs and taste preferences. These Spinach and Feta Stuffed Mushrooms are a delicious and nutritious snack or appetizer that's perfect for entertaining or enjoying on their own. Enjoy!

CHOCOLATE BANANA PROTEIN SMOOTHIE

Ingredients:

- 1 ripe banana
- 1 cup of unsweetened almond milk (or any milk of your choice)
- 1 scoop of chocolate protein powder
- 1 tablespoon of unsweetened cocoa powder
- 1 tablespoon of almond butter or peanut butter
- 1/2 teaspoon of vanilla extract
- Optional: ice cubes for a chilled smoothie

Instructions:

1. Peel the ripe banana and break it into chunks.
2. In a blender, combine the banana chunks, almond milk, chocolate protein powder, cocoa powder, almond butter or peanut butter, and vanilla extract.
3. Optional: Add a few ice cubes if you prefer a chilled smoothie.
4. Blend on high speed until all the ingredients

are well combined and the smoothie is creamy and smooth.

5. If the smoothie is too thick, add more almond milk. If it's too thin, add more ice or protein powder.
6. Pour the smoothie into a glass and enjoy immediately.

Macronutrient Breakdown:
- Banana provides natural sugars, carbs, and fiber.
- Almond milk offers a low-calorie base with minimal carbs and fats.
- Chocolate protein powder adds protein and enhances the chocolate flavor.
- Cocoa powder provides a rich chocolate taste with minimal impact on macros.
- Almond butter or peanut butter adds healthy fats and a creamy texture.

You can adjust the quantities to fit your personal macronutrient needs and taste preferences. This Chocolate Banana Protein Smoothie is a delicious and satisfying snack that's packed with protein, nutrients, and a rich chocolate flavor. It's perfect for a post-workout boost or as a sweet treat. Enjoy!

TURKEY MEATBALLS WITH GREEK YOGURT DIPPING SAUCE

Ingredients:

For the meatballs:

- 1 pound of lean ground turkey
- 1/4 cup of breadcrumbs (or almond meal for a gluten-free option)
- 1/4 cup of grated Parmesan cheese
- 1/4 cup of finely chopped onion
- 2 cloves of garlic, minced
- 1 teaspoon of dried oregano
- 1 teaspoon of dried basil
- 1/2 teaspoon of salt
- 1/4 teaspoon of black pepper
- Cooking spray or olive oil

For the dipping sauce:

- 1/2 cup of plain Greek yogurt
- 1 tablespoon of fresh lemon juice

- 1 tablespoon of chopped fresh dill
- 1/2 teaspoon of garlic powder
- Salt and pepper to taste

Instructions:

1. Preheat your oven to 400°F (200°C) and line a baking sheet with parchment paper.
2. In a large bowl, combine the ground turkey, breadcrumbs, grated Parmesan cheese, finely chopped onion, minced garlic, dried oregano, dried basil, salt, and black pepper. Mix well until all the ingredients are evenly incorporated.
3. Roll the turkey mixture into meatballs, approximately 1-2 inches in diameter, and place them on the prepared baking sheet.
4. Lightly spray the meatballs with cooking spray or brush them with a small amount of olive oil.
5. Bake for 15-20 minutes, or until the meatballs are cooked through and lightly browned.
6. While the meatballs are baking, prepare the Greek yogurt dipping sauce. In a small bowl, combine the plain Greek yogurt, fresh lemon juice, chopped fresh dill, garlic powder, salt, and pepper. Mix well until smooth and creamy.
7. Serve the turkey meatballs with the Greek yogurt dipping sauce on the side.

Macronutrient Breakdown:

- Lean ground turkey is a great source of protein with lower fat content compared to other meats.
- Breadcrumbs (or almond meal) add a small amount of carbs and help bind the meatballs.
- Parmesan cheese offers a bit of protein and flavor.
- Onion and garlic provide additional flavor without significant impact on macros.
- Greek yogurt adds protein and a creamy texture to the dipping sauce.
- Lemon juice, fresh dill, garlic powder, salt, and pepper enhance the flavor without adding excessive macros.

You can adjust the quantities and seasonings to fit your personal macronutrient needs and taste preferences. These Turkey Meatballs with Greek Yogurt Dipping Sauce are a protein-packed and flavorful snack that's perfect for satisfying your cravings. Enjoy them as an appetizer or as a protein boost throughout the day!

BAKED BUFFALO CAULIFLOWER BITES

Ingredients:
- 1 head of cauliflower, cut into florets
- 1/2 cup of whole wheat flour (or gluten-free flour of your choice)
- 1/2 cup of unsweetened almond milk (or any milk of your choice)
- 1 teaspoon of garlic powder
- 1/2 teaspoon of paprika
- 1/4 teaspoon of salt
- 1/4 teaspoon of black pepper
- 1/4 cup of hot sauce (such as Frank's RedHot or your favorite brand)
- 2 tablespoons of melted butter or olive oil
- Optional: Ranch or blue cheese dressing for dipping

Instructions:
1. Preheat your oven to 450°F (230°C) and line a baking sheet with parchment paper.
2. In a large bowl, whisk together the whole

wheat flour, almond milk, garlic powder, paprika, salt, and black pepper until you have a smooth batter.

3. Dip each cauliflower floret into the batter, coating it evenly, and let any excess batter drip off.

4. Place the coated cauliflower florets in a single layer on the prepared baking sheet.

5. Bake for 20-25 minutes, or until the cauliflower is tender and golden brown.

6. While the cauliflower is baking, in a separate bowl, mix together the hot sauce and melted butter or olive oil.

7. Remove the cauliflower from the oven and carefully toss it in the hot sauce mixture until coated.

8. Return the coated cauliflower to the baking sheet and bake for an additional 5 minutes to allow the sauce to penetrate and slightly caramelize.

9. Remove from the oven and let the buffalo cauliflower bites cool for a few minutes before serving.

10. Serve the buffalo cauliflower bites with ranch or blue cheese dressing on the side for dipping.

Macronutrient Breakdown:

- Cauliflower is low in calories and provides fiber, vitamins, and minerals.
- Whole wheat flour adds complex carbs and

some protein.

- Almond milk offers a low-calorie base with minimal carbs and fats.
- Hot sauce provides flavor without significant impact on macros.
- Butter or olive oil adds a touch of healthy fats and richness.
- Ranch or blue cheese dressing (if using) contributes additional flavor and texture.

You can adjust the quantities and choice of dipping sauce to fit your personal macronutrient needs and taste preferences. These Baked Buffalo Cauliflower Bites are a delicious and nutritious alternative to traditional buffalo wings. They offer a spicy kick and a satisfying crunch. Enjoy them as a game-day snack or a guilt-free appetizer!

AVOCADO EGG SALAD LETTUCE WRAPS

Ingredients:

- 4 hard-boiled eggs, peeled and chopped
- 1 ripe avocado, pitted and mashed
- 2 tablespoons of Greek yogurt (or mayonnaise)
- 1 tablespoon of Dijon mustard
- 1 tablespoon of fresh lemon juice
- 2 tablespoons of finely chopped red onion
- 2 tablespoons of chopped fresh dill (or any fresh herbs you prefer)
- Salt and pepper to taste
- 4 large lettuce leaves (such as romaine or butter lettuce)
- Optional: Sliced cherry tomatoes and cucumber for added freshness

Instructions:

1. In a bowl, combine the chopped hard-boiled eggs, mashed avocado, Greek yogurt (or mayonnaise), Dijon mustard, fresh lemon juice, red onion, chopped fresh dill, salt, and

pepper. Mix well until all the ingredients are thoroughly combined.

2. Lay out the large lettuce leaves on a clean surface.
3. Spoon the avocado egg salad mixture onto each lettuce leaf, dividing it equally among them.
4. If desired, add sliced cherry tomatoes and cucumber on top of the avocado egg salad mixture for added freshness.
5. Gently roll up each lettuce leaf to form a wrap, securing it with toothpicks if needed.
6. Serve the avocado egg salad lettuce wraps immediately.

Macronutrient Breakdown:
- Hard-boiled eggs provide protein and healthy fats.
- Avocado offers healthy fats and a creamy texture.
- Greek yogurt (or mayonnaise) adds creaminess and a touch of protein.
- Dijon mustard and fresh lemon juice add tanginess and flavor.
- Red onion and fresh dill (or herbs) enhance the taste without significant macros.
- Lettuce leaves provide a low-calorie and refreshing base.
- Optional cherry tomatoes and cucumber offer vitamins, minerals, and fiber.

You can adjust the quantities and choice of veggies

to fit your personal macronutrient needs and taste preferences. These Avocado Egg Salad Lettuce Wraps are a light and satisfying snack that's packed with protein and healthy fats. Enjoy them as a refreshing lunch option or a tasty afternoon pick-me-up!

ALMOND BUTTER PROTEIN BALLS

Ingredients:

- 1 cup of rolled oats
- 1/2 cup of almond butter
- 1/4 cup of honey or maple syrup
- 1/4 cup of chocolate protein powder
- 2 tablespoons of ground flaxseed
- 2 tablespoons of mini chocolate chips (optional)
- 1 teaspoon of vanilla extract
- Pinch of salt

Instructions:

1. In a large bowl, combine the rolled oats, almond butter, honey or maple syrup, chocolate protein powder, ground flaxseed, mini chocolate chips (if using), vanilla extract, and salt. Mix well until all the ingredients are thoroughly combined.
2. Place the mixture in the refrigerator for about 30 minutes to allow it to firm up.
3. After chilling, remove the mixture from the refrigerator and roll it into small balls,

about 1 inch in diameter.

4. Optional: If desired, roll the protein balls in additional ground flaxseed or mini chocolate chips for coating.
5. Place the almond butter protein balls on a plate or baking sheet lined with parchment paper.
6. Refrigerate the protein balls for at least 1 hour, or until firm.
7. Once chilled, transfer the protein balls to an airtight container and store them in the refrigerator.

Macronutrient Breakdown:
- Rolled oats provide complex carbs and fiber.
- Almond butter offers healthy fats and a bit of protein.
- Honey or maple syrup adds sweetness and carbs.
- Chocolate protein powder boosts the protein content.
- Ground flaxseed provides additional fiber and healthy fats.
- Mini chocolate chips (if using) add a touch of sweetness and flavor.

You can adjust the quantities and sweetness level to fit your personal macronutrient needs and taste preferences. These Almond Butter Protein Balls are a convenient and tasty snack that's packed with protein and fiber. They're perfect for an on-the-go energy boost or a post-workout recovery snack.

Enjoy!

CAPRESE STUFFED AVOCADO

Ingredients:

- 2 ripe avocados, halved and pitted
- 1 cup of cherry tomatoes, halved
- 4 ounces of fresh mozzarella cheese, diced
- 1/4 cup of fresh basil leaves, torn
- 1 tablespoon of balsamic glaze or balsamic reduction
- Salt and pepper to taste

Instructions:

1. Scoop out some of the flesh from each avocado half, creating a hollow space for the stuffing. Reserve the scooped-out flesh for another use or enjoy it as a snack.
2. In a bowl, combine the cherry tomatoes, fresh mozzarella cheese, and torn basil leaves.
3. Gently toss the mixture to evenly distribute the ingredients.
4. Spoon the tomato, mozzarella, and basil

    mixture into each avocado half, filling them generously.

5. Drizzle the stuffed avocados with balsamic glaze or balsamic reduction.
6. Season with salt and pepper to taste.
7. Serve the Caprese Stuffed Avocado immediately.

Macronutrient Breakdown:

- Avocado offers healthy fats, vitamins, and minerals.
- Cherry tomatoes provide vitamins, minerals, and fiber.
- Fresh mozzarella cheese adds protein and a creamy texture.
- Fresh basil leaves add flavor and antioxidants.
- Balsamic glaze or balsamic reduction provides tanginess and minimal impact on macros.
- Salt and pepper enhance taste with minimal macros.

You can adjust the quantities and choice of ingredients to fit your personal macronutrient needs and taste preferences. These Caprese Stuffed Avocados are a refreshing and nutrient-dense snack that combines the creaminess of avocado with the vibrant flavors of tomatoes, mozzarella, and basil. They're perfect for a quick appetizer or a light meal. Enjoy!

CHICKPEA SALAD LETTUCE WRAPS

Ingredients:

- 1 can (15 ounces) of chickpeas, drained and rinsed
- 1/4 cup of diced red onion
- 1/4 cup of diced cucumber
- 1/4 cup of diced bell pepper (any color)
- 2 tablespoons of chopped fresh parsley
- 2 tablespoons of lemon juice
- 2 tablespoons of olive oil
- 1 teaspoon of Dijon mustard
- Salt and pepper to taste
- 4 large lettuce leaves (such as butter lettuce or romaine)

Instructions:

1. In a bowl, lightly mash the chickpeas using a fork or potato masher, leaving some texture.
2. Add the diced red onion, cucumber, bell pepper, chopped fresh parsley, lemon juice, olive oil, Dijon mustard, salt, and pepper to the mashed chickpeas.

3. Mix well until all the ingredients are thoroughly combined and the flavors are evenly distributed.
4. Taste and adjust the seasonings if needed.
5. Lay out the large lettuce leaves on a clean surface.
6. Spoon the chickpea salad mixture onto each lettuce leaf, dividing it equally among them.
7. Gently roll up each lettuce leaf to form a wrap.
8. Secure the wraps with toothpicks if desired.
9. Serve the chickpea salad lettuce wraps immediately.

Macronutrient Breakdown:
- Chickpeas provide plant-based protein, fiber, and complex carbs.
- Red onion, cucumber, and bell pepper offer vitamins, minerals, and fiber.
- Fresh parsley adds flavor and antioxidants.
- Lemon juice, olive oil, and Dijon mustard enhance the taste without significant macros.
- Lettuce leaves provide a low-calorie and refreshing base.

You can adjust the quantities and choice of veggies to fit your personal macronutrient needs and taste preferences. These Chickpea Salad Lettuce Wraps are a protein-rich and satisfying snack that's perfect for a light lunch or a quick and nutritious meal on the go. Enjoy!

SWEET POTATO TOAST WITH AVOCADO AND EGG

Ingredients:

- 1 large sweet potato, sliced into 1/2-inch thick rounds
- 1 ripe avocado
- 2 large eggs
- Salt and pepper to taste
- Optional toppings: crushed red pepper flakes, fresh herbs, or hot sauce

Instructions:

1. Preheat your oven to 400°F (200°C) and line a baking sheet with parchment paper.
2. Place the sweet potato slices on the prepared baking sheet and bake for about 15-20 minutes, or until the sweet potato is tender.
3. While the sweet potato is baking, cut the

avocado in half, remove the pit, and scoop the flesh into a bowl. Mash the avocado with a fork until smooth. Season with salt and pepper to taste.

4. In a non-stick skillet, fry the eggs to your desired doneness (such as over-easy or sunny-side-up). Season with salt and pepper.
5. Once the sweet potato rounds are cooked, remove them from the oven and let them cool slightly.
6. Spread a generous amount of mashed avocado on each sweet potato round.
7. Top each round with a fried egg.
8. Optional: Sprinkle with crushed red pepper flakes, fresh herbs, or add a drizzle of hot sauce for added flavor and heat.
9. Serve the Sweet Potato Toast with Avocado and Egg immediately.

Macronutrient Breakdown:
- Sweet potatoes provide complex carbs, fiber, and vitamins.
- Avocado offers healthy fats and fiber.
- Eggs provide protein and healthy fats.
- Salt and pepper enhance taste with minimal macros.
- Optional toppings add flavor without significant macros.

You can adjust the quantities and choice of toppings to fit your personal macronutrient needs and taste preferences. These Sweet Potato Toast with Avocado and Egg slices are a satisfying and nutritious snack or light meal that's packed with a balance of carbs, healthy fats, and protein. Enjoy!

GREEK YOGURT BERRY BARK

Ingredients:
- 1 cup of plain Greek yogurt
- 2 tablespoons of honey or maple syrup
- 1/2 teaspoon of vanilla extract
- 1 cup of mixed berries (such as strawberries, blueberries, and raspberries)
- 2 tablespoons of chopped nuts (such as almonds or walnuts)
- 2 tablespoons of unsweetened shredded coconut

Instructions:
1. In a bowl, mix together the Greek yogurt, honey or maple syrup, and vanilla extract until well combined.
2. Line a baking sheet with parchment paper.
3. Pour the Greek yogurt mixture onto the prepared baking sheet, spreading it out evenly with a spatula to create a thin layer.
4. Sprinkle the mixed berries, chopped nuts, and shredded coconut over the Greek yogurt layer, pressing them down gently.

5. Place the baking sheet in the freezer and let it freeze for at least 2-3 hours, or until firm.
6. Once frozen, remove the Greek yogurt berry bark from the baking sheet and break it into smaller pieces using your hands or a knife.
7. Serve the Greek Yogurt Berry Bark immediately or store it in an airtight container in the freezer.

Macronutrient Breakdown:
- Greek yogurt provides protein, calcium, and probiotics.
- Honey or maple syrup adds natural sweetness and carbs.
- Vanilla extract enhances the flavor without significant macros.
- Mixed berries offer vitamins, minerals, and fiber.
- Chopped nuts provide healthy fats and a satisfying crunch.
- Unsweetened shredded coconut adds flavor and texture.

You can adjust the quantities and choice of berries and nuts to fit your personal macronutrient needs and taste preferences. This Greek Yogurt Berry Bark is a refreshing and nutritious snack that's perfect for satisfying your sweet tooth while providing a balance of protein, carbs, and healthy fats. Enjoy!

BAKED EGGPLANT PARMESAN BITES

Ingredients:

- 1 medium eggplant, sliced into 1/2-inch thick rounds
- 1 cup of whole wheat breadcrumbs (or almond flour for a gluten-free option)
- 1/2 cup of grated Parmesan cheese
- 2 large eggs, beaten
- 1 teaspoon of dried Italian seasoning
- 1/2 teaspoon of garlic powder
- 1/2 teaspoon of onion powder
- 1/4 teaspoon of salt
- Cooking spray or olive oil

For the dipping sauce:

- 1 cup of marinara sauce
- Optional: Fresh basil leaves for garnish

Instructions:

1. Preheat your oven to 400°F (200°C) and line a baking sheet with parchment paper.
2. In a shallow dish, combine the whole wheat breadcrumbs (or almond flour), grated

Parmesan cheese, dried Italian seasoning, garlic powder, onion powder, and salt.

3. Dip each eggplant round into the beaten eggs, allowing any excess to drip off.
4. Coat the eggplant round in the breadcrumb mixture, pressing it down gently to adhere.
5. Place the coated eggplant rounds on the prepared baking sheet.
6. Lightly spray the tops of the eggplant rounds with cooking spray or brush them with a small amount of olive oil.
7. Bake for 20-25 minutes, or until the eggplant is tender and the coating is golden brown and crispy.
8. While the eggplant bites are baking, warm up the marinara sauce in a small saucepan over low heat.
9. Once the eggplant bites are done, remove them from the oven and let them cool for a few minutes.
10. Serve the Baked Eggplant Parmesan Bites with the warm marinara sauce for dipping.
11. Optional: Garnish with fresh basil leaves for added flavor and presentation.

Macronutrient Breakdown:

- Eggplant provides low calories and carbs with fiber and antioxidants.
- Whole wheat breadcrumbs (or almond flour) add complex carbs and fiber.

- Grated Parmesan cheese offers protein and flavor.
- Eggs provide protein and healthy fats.
- Dried Italian seasoning, garlic powder, onion powder, and salt add flavor without excessive macros.
- Marinara sauce adds minimal macros and is rich in flavor.

You can adjust the quantities and choice of coating to fit your personal macronutrient needs and taste preferences. These Baked Eggplant Parmesan Bites are a healthier twist on the classic Italian dish, offering a crispy texture and a burst of flavor. Enjoy them as a delicious appetizer or a satisfying snack!

CAULIFLOWER HUMMUS

Ingredients:

- 1 small head of cauliflower, cut into florets
- 2 cloves of garlic, minced
- 2 tablespoons of tahini
- 2 tablespoons of lemon juice
- 1 tablespoon of olive oil
- 1/2 teaspoon of ground cumin
- 1/4 teaspoon of paprika
- Salt and pepper to taste
- Optional toppings: drizzle of olive oil, sprinkle of paprika, chopped parsley

Instructions:

1. Steam or boil the cauliflower florets until they are tender. Drain and let them cool slightly.
2. In a food processor, combine the steamed cauliflower, minced garlic, tahini, lemon juice, olive oil, ground cumin, paprika, salt, and pepper.
3. Process the mixture until smooth and creamy, scraping down the sides of the food

    processor as needed.
4. Taste and adjust the seasonings if needed.
5. Transfer the cauliflower hummus to a serving dish.
6. Optional: Drizzle with olive oil, sprinkle with paprika, and garnish with chopped parsley for added flavor and presentation.
7. Serve the Cauliflower Hummus with your favorite vegetables, whole grain crackers, or as a spread in sandwiches and wraps.

Macronutrient Breakdown:
- Cauliflower is low in calories and carbs while providing fiber, vitamins, and minerals.
- Garlic adds flavor and potential health benefits.
- Tahini offers healthy fats and a creamy texture.
- Lemon juice provides a tangy taste and a boost of vitamin C.
- Olive oil adds healthy fats and richness.
- Ground cumin and paprika enhance the flavor without excessive macros.
- Salt and pepper enhance taste with minimal macros.

You can adjust the quantities and choice of toppings to fit your personal macronutrient needs and taste preferences. This Cauliflower Hummus is a delicious and nutritious alternative to traditional chickpea hummus. It's perfect for dipping vegetables, spreading on toast, or adding flavor to your favorite dishes. Enjoy!

TURKEY AND QUINOA STUFFED BELL PEPPERS

Ingredients:

- 4 bell peppers (any color)
- 1 cup of cooked quinoa
- 1/2 pound of lean ground turkey
- 1/4 cup of diced onion
- 1/4 cup of diced bell pepper (any color)
- 1 clove of garlic, minced
- 1/4 cup of tomato sauce
- 1/2 teaspoon of dried basil
- 1/2 teaspoon of dried oregano
- 1/4 teaspoon of paprika
- Salt and pepper to taste
- Optional: Shredded cheese for topping

Instructions:

1. Preheat your oven to 375°F (190°C).
2. Cut off the tops of the bell peppers and remove the seeds and membranes from the inside.
3. In a large skillet, cook the ground turkey

over medium heat until browned and cooked through.

4. Add the diced onion, diced bell pepper, and minced garlic to the skillet with the cooked turkey. Sauté for a few minutes until the vegetables have softened.
5. Stir in the cooked quinoa, tomato sauce, dried basil, dried oregano, paprika, salt, and pepper. Cook for a few more minutes to allow the flavors to meld together.
6. Fill each bell pepper with the turkey and quinoa mixture, packing it in tightly.
7. Optional: Sprinkle shredded cheese on top of each stuffed bell pepper.
8. Place the stuffed bell peppers in a baking dish or on a baking sheet.
9. Bake for 25-30 minutes, or until the bell peppers are tender and the filling is heated through.
10. Remove from the oven and let the stuffed bell peppers cool for a few minutes before serving.

Macronutrient Breakdown:
- Bell peppers provide low calories, carbs, and high vitamin content.
- Quinoa offers complex carbs, protein, and fiber.
- Lean ground turkey adds protein and minimal fat.
- Onion, bell pepper, and garlic provide flavor without significant macros.

- Tomato sauce enhances taste with minimal macros.
- Dried basil, dried oregano, paprika, salt, and pepper add flavor without excessive macros.
- Optional shredded cheese adds a touch of creaminess and protein.

You can adjust the quantities and choice of seasonings to fit your personal macronutrient needs and taste preferences. These Turkey and Quinoa Stuffed Bell Peppers are a satisfying and nutritious snack or light meal that's packed with protein, complex carbs, and vegetables. Enjoy them as a tasty lunch option or a delicious dinner!

SPICY SHRIMP LETTUCE WRAPS

Ingredients:
- 1 pound of shrimp, peeled and deveined
- 2 tablespoons of low-sodium soy sauce
- 1 tablespoon of sriracha sauce (adjust for desired spice level)
- 1 tablespoon of honey or maple syrup
- 1 tablespoon of lime juice
- 1 teaspoon of minced garlic
- 1 teaspoon of grated fresh ginger
- 1 tablespoon of olive oil
- Salt and pepper to taste
- 8 large lettuce leaves (such as butter lettuce or romaine)
- Optional toppings: sliced cucumbers, shredded carrots, chopped cilantro

Instructions:
1. In a bowl, combine the low-sodium soy sauce, sriracha sauce, honey or maple syrup, lime juice, minced garlic, grated fresh ginger, olive oil, salt, and pepper. Mix well to create a marinade.

2. Add the shrimp to the marinade and toss to coat them evenly. Let the shrimp marinate for about 15 minutes.
3. Heat a non-stick skillet over medium heat.
4. Add the marinated shrimp to the skillet, along with any remaining marinade.
5. Cook the shrimp for 2-3 minutes per side, or until they are pink and cooked through.
6. Remove the cooked shrimp from the skillet and let them cool slightly.
7. Lay out the large lettuce leaves on a clean surface.
8. Place a few shrimp on each lettuce leaf, dividing them equally.
9. Optional: Add sliced cucumbers, shredded carrots, and chopped cilantro on top of the shrimp for added freshness and crunch.
10. Gently roll up each lettuce leaf to form a wrap.
11. Serve the Spicy Shrimp Lettuce Wraps immediately.

Macronutrient Breakdown:
- Shrimp provides lean protein with minimal carbs and fat.
- Low-sodium soy sauce adds flavor with minimal macros.
- Sriracha sauce provides heat and flavor without significant macros.
- Honey or maple syrup adds sweetness and carbs.

- Lime juice adds tanginess and vitamin C.
- Garlic and ginger enhance the taste without excessive macros.
- Olive oil offers healthy fats.
- Lettuce leaves provide a low-calorie and refreshing base.
- Optional toppings add crunch, vitamins, and minerals.

You can adjust the quantities and choice of toppings to fit your personal macronutrient needs and taste preferences. These Spicy Shrimp Lettuce Wraps are a flavorful and protein-packed snack that's perfect for a light lunch or a quick and nutritious meal. Enjoy!

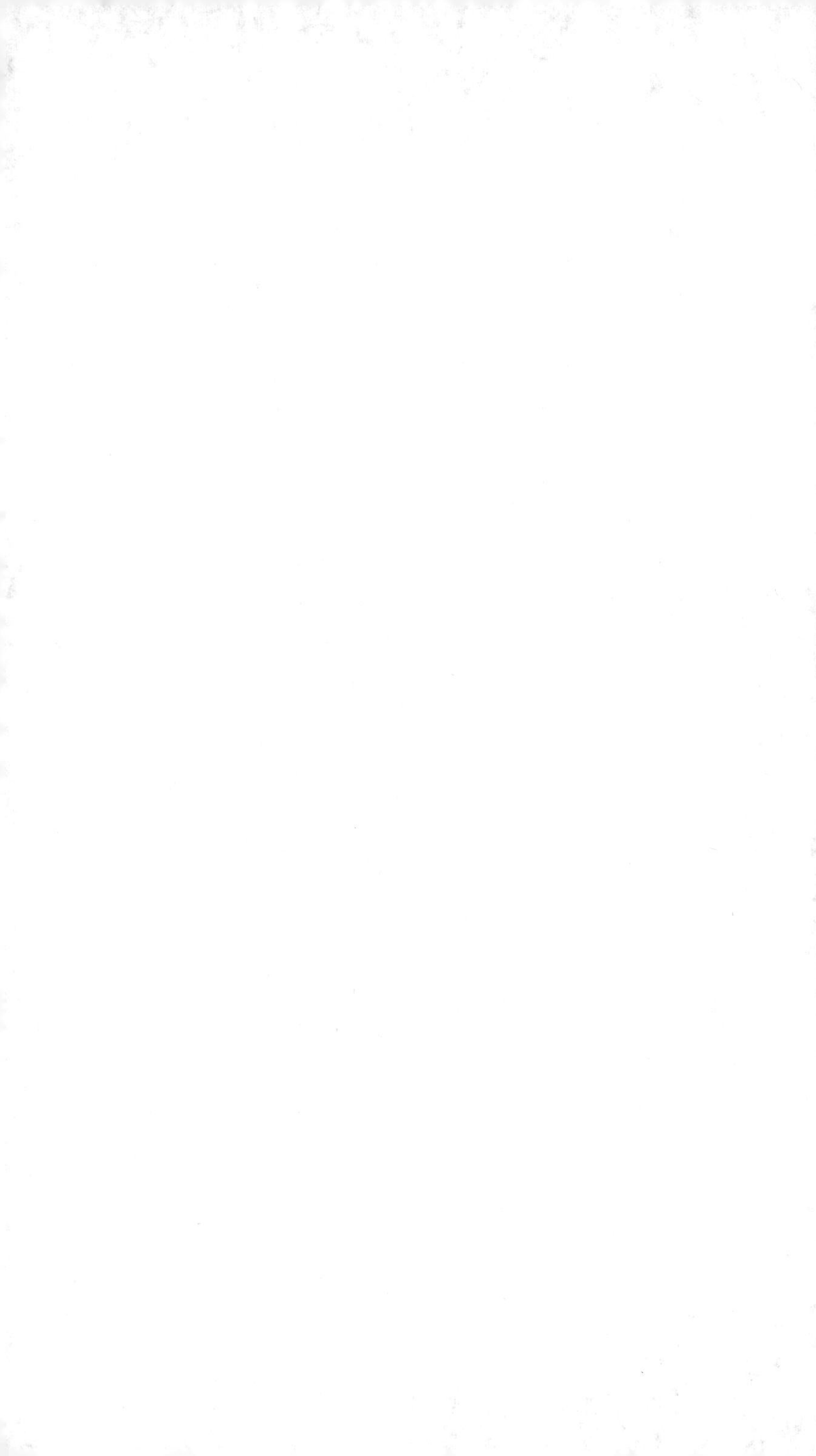

www.ingramcontent.com/pod-product-compliance
Lightning Source LLC
Chambersburg PA
CBHW061650250726

48659CB00004B/1438